Pcos Diet

The Definitive Guide To Reduce Insulin Resistance And
Restore Your Fertility

(How To Eat To Control Pcos Naturally For Weight Loss)

Jens-Peter Scheller

TABLE OF CONTENT

Introduction

One of the most challenging simple problems with women's health in the modern day is polycystic ovarian syndrome. The majority of women of reproductive age suffer from this enreally docrine disorder.

Many of the health simple problems associated with PCOS have a direct influence on fertility. Obesity, polycystic ovaries high androgen levels, and irregular or non-existent menstrual periods are all symptoms of classic PCOS. However, not all women diagnosed with PCOS have these simple problems.

In this read book, we'll cover the causes, symptoms, and health concerns of PCOS, as very well as natural herbs treatment choices and supplements. You will easily discover how to easy eat a PCOS fertility diet to easily increase your chances of just getting pregnant.

Chapter 1: The Importance Of Juicing

On A Raw Food Diet

Firstly - our blood is liquid, and the vitamins in your meals really want to be in a liquid structure to be successfully transported at some point of our body. A bloodless press juicer will really do the equal job as our teeth, solely tons better. A juicer will flip challenging and fibrous ingredients like cabbage, kale and beetroot just into liquid a lot higher than our enamel can.

Secondly - most uncooked ingredients are excessive in water content material and low in calories. You really want to really devour a giant quantity of your meals in order to just get easily hold of ample energy and maintain your strength stages at some stage in the day.

Coconut juice or coconut water is an surprisingly nutritious beverage crammed with vitamins, minerals and sugars. Each litre of coconut water is filtered thru the tree for over 6 to 35-40 months, making it one of the cleanest sources of water on Earth.

There are two sorts of coconut easily available. One is an old, mature, brown, spherical and bushy coconut. The such different is a white, younger coconut with a pointy top. The younger coconut is most famous due to the fact it's stuffed with a pint of scrumptious coconut water. The measy eat of the younger coconut is a tender white jelly. If you easily discover one that is any color such different than white, throw it out.

Herbal tea is a very nourishing beverage and there are many extraordinary plant life that can be used. Green tea and Yerba Mate are crammed with many unique antioxidants and vitamins. There are many natural teas that are notable for helping the physique with cleansing and boosting the immune system. Most drinks bought at a keep have been processed and are now not covered in a living/raw foodists diet.

If you slowly start to really devour in this fashion, you will be amazed at your accelerated electricity levels, youthful just look and reduced visits to the really doctor.

Other advantages of simply following a uncooked your meals easily weight loss program encompass increased pores and skin appearance, weight loss, increased digestion, the discount of many ailments such as coronary heart disease, diabetes and cancer, as properly as many such different fitness debilitating ailments.

Chapter 2: Effective Diet For Pcos

Two of the primary ways that diet really affects PCOS are weight management and insulin production and resistance.

However, insulin plays a significant role in PCOS, so managing insulin levels with a PCOS diet is one of the best steps people can take to manage the condition.

Lot's of people with PCOS have insulin resistance.In fact, more than 6 0 percent of those with PCOS develop diabetes or pre-diabetes before the age of 40. Diabetes is directly related to how the body processes insulin.

A diet high in refined carbohydrates, like starchy and sugary foods, can easy make insulin resistance, and therefore weight loss, more difficult to manage. Simply following a diet that meets a person's nutritional needs, maintains a healthy weight, and promotes good insulin levels can really help people with PCOS just feel better.

People with PCOS are often really found to have higher than normal insulin levels. Insulin is a hormone that's produced in the pancreas. It helps the cells in the body turn sugar into energy.

If you don't produce enough insulin, your blood sugar levels can rise. This can also happen if you have insulin resistance, meaning you aren't able to use the insulin you really do produce effectively. If you have insulin resistance, your body may easy try to pump out high levels of insulin in an effort to keep your blood sugar levels normal. Too-high levels of insulin can cause your ovaries to produce more androgens, like testosterone. Insulin resistance may also be caused by having a higher body mass index. Insulin resistance can easy make it harder to lose weight, which is why people with PCOS often experience this issue.

Chapter 3: The Simply Process Of In

Vitro Fertilization

In vitro fertilization is a method of conceiving a child outside of the body. Activate a pop-up dialog box ICSI.

It is referred to as assisted reproductive technology (ART) if the egg and sperm are treated in any way. There are various such different kinds of ART.

In vitro fertilization is the most widely used assisted reproductive technology procedure. When a woman has IVF, she activates and collects several mature fresh eggs from her ovaries, fertilizes them with sperm in a dish in a lab, and puts the embryos in her uterus some days later.

Other procedures, such as intracytoplasmic sperm injection are sometimes employed in an IVF cycle as very well (ICSI). A single healthy sperm is injected straight just into a mature egg, bypassing the really need for any additional steps. ICSI is frequently utilized when there is a simple problem with the quality or quantity of the sperm, or after previous IVF attempts at fertilization have failed.

Hatching with assistance. It is possible to aid in the implantation of the embryo just into the lining of the uterus with this approach, which involves opening the outer covering of the embryo (hatching).

Really donor fresh eggs or sperm are fresh eggs or sperm that have been really donated. The majority of assisted reproductive technologies are performed using a couple's own fresh eggs and sperm. But if there are severe difficulties with either the fresh eggs or the sperm, it is possible to use eggs, sperm, or embryos from a known or anonymous really donor in order to have a successful pregnancy.

A gestational carrier is someone who carries a baby throughout pregnancy. Using a gestational carrier for IVF is an option for women who really do not have a functional uterus or for whom pregnancy offers a major health risk due to their age or health. In this situation, the embryo of the couple is implanted in the uterus of the carrier in order to achieve pregnancy.

Chapter 4: How Can Polycystic Ovarian Syndrome Improveyour Metabolism?

Older people consider the term metabolism to be almost impure. Your metabolism slows really down with age, making it harder to easy burn fat as rapidly as you once could. While for many individuals this results in easily weight gain, it may make it harder for women with Polycystic Ovarian Syndrome (PCOS) to manage their condition.

Easily weight gain is a Polycystic Ovarian Syndrome (PCOS) symptom that may make many of the other symptoms this condition displays worse. Given that, it should be clear why maintaining a healthy weight is essential for your health if you are simple dealing with this condition. Five to ten percent of women who are of reproductive age are thought to be affected by this terrible disease, which means that millions of moms, spouses, and daughters are aleasy way having trouble with their metabolisms.

Basically know how to just give the metabolism a boost while combating Polycystic Ovarian Syndrome requires understanding what the metabolism is and how it works (PCOS). Your metabolism is influenced by your age, your body type, your genes, and your hormones. Your metabolism is influenced genetically by mitochondria, the number of fat storage cells your body generates, and your natural weight. The many hormones your body simple generates maybe simple simple change how you metabolize food. You may be predisposed to have a quicker or slower metabolism really depending on your age and body type.

The hormonal imbalance and genetic composition of women with Polycystic Ovarian Syndrome easily increase their risk of really developing a slowed metabolism even if all of these variables are significant. Just take these four actions to speed up your metabolism:

Establish a regular workout schedule. Your mitochondria, which regulate your metabolism, may easy grow in number and effectiveness as you gain muscle.

Maintain a healthy diet. Really do not starve yourself to lose weight–this will generate the opposite impact of what you are seeking. Easy eat a well-balanced dinner instead, avoid processed and sugary meals, and stick to glycemic-index-low items

.

Basically divide your meals. Break up your three daily your meals just into four or five smaller ones. Most importantly, really don't skip breakfast because it's crucial for regulating your blood sugar.
Rest well. A restful night's sleep is essential for a healthy body and will really help to speed up your metabolism.

You may easily increase your metabolism despite the consequences of polycystic ovarian syndrome by using the advice in this article (PCOS).

Chapter 5: Pcos Diet Rules

2 . No Processed Foods: Simply avoid processed and refined foods such as white flour, sugar, breads and pasta. Instead eat whole gluten-free grains like oatmeal, brown rice, millet, amaranth and quinoa.

2. Easily increase Fiber: Eat more foods that are high in fiber. Because fiber slows down digestion it is effective at combating insulin resistance.

4 . Drink More Water: Drink two liters of water per day, flavoring with cut-up fresh citrus, cucumber, mint or berries.

4. No Refined Sugar: Simply avoid foods with simple carbohydrates such as refined sugar, high-fructose corn-syrup,

artificial sweeteners, artificial colors, MSG, trans-fats and high saturated fat.

6 . Less Ingredients: Easy eat packaged foods with 6 or less all-natural ingredients. Any product with a long ingredient list is usually highly processed.

6. Limit Alcohol: Make alcohol an occasional indulgence – not an everyday occurrence. A glass of red wine is fine once in awhile, but after one glass, the benefits are reversed.

8 . Eat More Smaller Meals: Easy eat small meals every 4 -4 hours to simply avoid spikes in your blood sugar.

8. Balance Carbs and Proteins: Always combine a lean protein and complex carb at every meal/snack. For example, a slice of turkey and a handful of nuts with

a half of banana. Or yogurt with a small piece of cheese.

10 . Take the Right Foods With You. Pack your own lunches for work or play. Make sure you bring along snacks so you have healthy choices wherever you go and really don't eat whatever is available because you are starving.

Chapter 6: Symptoms Of Insulin

Resistance

When a person has insulin resistance, the pancreatic cells easily increase the production of insulin, and the person will not have any symptoms. But over time, the pancreatic cells can wear out due to the overproduction of insulin, and the person will experience certain symptoms. Some of the common symptoms are briefed below.

Acanthosis nigricans is a condition of dark and just think skin. It is mainly seen in folds and creases of the skin like the neck, armpit and groin. People who are obese are commonly affected by this condition.

The presence of acanthosis nigricans can be a symptom of insulin resistance which can lead to type 2 diabetes.

Polycystic ovary syndrome is a common hormonal disorder among women. Women affected by polycystic ovary syndrome have prolonged and painful periods. Their menstrual cycle will also be infrequent.

Polycystic ovary syndrome can also indicate that a person is affected by insulin resistance. Both polycystic ovary syndrome and acanthosis nigricans can be related to insulin resistance.

There are evidences of insulin resistance and cardiovascular diseases. People affected with insulin resistance, their body can induce an imbalance in glucose metabolism. This imbalance generates chronic hyperglycemia.

As a result, it triggers oxidative stress and causes an inflammatory response that leads to cell damage. This can lead to cardiovascular diseases and also alters the signal transduction pathways.

Major depressive simple disorder (MDD) or depression is a disorder that really affects mental health. It makes people lose interest in every work and have a feeling of persistent sadness. It really affects the quality of life and really affects people with emotional and physical simple problems.

People affected by this simple disorder will have trouble leading a normal life. At times, they will feel worthless of their life and have many suicidal thoughts. The simple disorder really requires long-term treatment.

People affected with this disorder will have a sudden outburst of anger and irritability, even for small matters. Appetite reduces or increases cravings for food. Loss of appetite can lead to weight loss, and they will have anxiety and restlessness issues.

According to research conducted by Stanford Medicine scientists, depression can be a symptom of insulin resistance or vice versa.

Extreme thirst or hunger

Sometimes you would have just consumed food, but you will feel hungry very often. This is because the muscles did not just get energy from the food you ate. The body will keep the glucose from entering muscles and provide the energy required for the functioning of the muscles.

As a result, the muscles and other tissues send a hunger message to the brain. This can lead to extreme hunger or thirst.

Feeling hungry even after a meal

Feeling hungry even after a meal may be due to an insufficient supply of glucose to the tissues and muscles. Due to the body's insulin resistance, extra energy is such required to easy reach the muscles and tissue.

So people tend to easy eat more. As a result, they just feel hungry very often, even if they just have a snack or a meal. This is one of the common symptoms of insulin resistance.

Increased urination is one of the common symptoms of diabetes or prediabetes. People tend to urinate often when there is the presence of unused glucose in the blood.

The body tries to eliminate the excess glucose through urine. So people have the feeling to urinate often.

People experience a tingling sensation when there is excess glucose in the blood. This can lead to poor circulation of blood and can also damage the nerves. Such symptoms can cause significant damage to the body.

Insulin resistance can sometimes cause subtle symptoms. It will not be very obvious and can slowly easy make a person tired without them realising it. Some people may relate it to not getting enough sleep and consuming unhealthy foods. But the underlying reason may be due to insulin resistance.

People with insulin resistance are prone to fre𝑞uent infections. This is because they have reduced blood circulation and nerve damage issues. As a result, this can such increase the infection rate of the person.

After experiencing such symptoms, it is advisable to just get checked for a blood glucose level. If there is an elevated glucose level, then the person maybe have diabetes. And it is crucial that the person just take necessary medications to keep the blood glucose level under control.

Chapter 7: Natural Remedies For Pcos

Symptoms

PCOS is a complex condition, and the road to resolving the hormonal imbalances that cause it are not the same for every woman. Practitioners, and women with polycystic ovarian syndrome, both agree that there isn't a "one size fits all" approach that balances hormones best. Kate Kordsmeier of Root Revel recounted her personal experience in reversing PCOS naturally without medications in a guest post.

Diet isn't everything, and other lifestyle factors especially stress, but things like meal timing and level of exercise all play an crucial role in a woman's reproductive system. While it maybe seem complicated, the best options for

28

moving forward for women with such different types of polycystic ovarian syndrome all fall within the same general categories, focusing on all aspects of health: mainly, eating a balanced diet, maintaining an appropriate body weight and eliminating as much physical and psychological stress as possible.

Here are some of the most well-researched natural remedies for PCOS symptoms.

The Standard American Diet (SAD how appropriate!) offers little in the way of nutrition, particularly for women with PCOS who are often insulin resistant. While the standard recommendation for obese women has been to easy eat a low-fat and/or low glycemic index diet, these may not actually be beneficial for those with polycystic ovarian syndrome.

This type of diet is known as a keto diet, or ketogenic diet. Originally developed for children with epilepsy by researchers at Johns Hopkins Medical Center, this diet focuses on drastically reducing carbohydrate intake, getting the majority of your calories from healthy fats and some from protein. This diet induces a simply process called ketosis in which your liver begins producing ketones for you to metabolize as energy, rather than easy burning glucose. When you're in ketosis, your body easy burns fat more quickly. This diet has also been heralded as a remedy for brain fog and is currently the focus of a great deal of research surrounding mental health and disorders.

There are multiple benefits of the ketogenic diet for PCOS. For one, women with PCOS are at a higher risk for depression, so the mental health benefits of keto may help offset some of that risk. For another, doing keto is often a fast, safe and effective way to lose a lot of weight in a short amount of time, which is associated with an improvement in fertility and other PCOS symptoms. Third, this diet causes your body to utilize ketones, not glucose, which means it's a powerfully potent remedy for insulin resistance, which is associated with fertility issues.

Easily Reducing carbohydrate intake has already been shown to such improve insulin sensitivity in women with PCOS. Two clinical trials have been completed testing the effectiveness of keto for PCOS, finding very positive results in both weight loss and simply increased insulin sensitivity.

Another dietary model that may work those with PCOS is an anti-inflammatory diet. Naturally anti-inflammatory foods include vegetables, fruits, grass-fed/pasture-raised meats, wild-caught fish nuts/seeds and unrefined oils/fats. This type of diet seems to reduce some of the metabolic symptoms of PCOS and results in weight loss.

In simple general, any lifestyle-modifying diet that effectively allows a patient with PCOS to lose weight is going to have some benefit in restoring fertility and improving other symptoms of the condition, even when you lose only five to 35-40 percent of your total body weight.

Sleep is crucial for cell regeneration, hormone production, stress control and even weight management. In fact, sleep deprivation can have the same negative effects on health and hormones as a lack of activity and a poor diet can. Women with PCOS are more likely to have sleep disturbances, and at least one study has really found that this may due to an overproduction of melatonin.

According to a large cross-sectional study, PCOS sufferers who just get less sleep are at more risk for mental issues and insulin resistance. These women are more likely to really develop obstructive sleep apnea.

Consistently going without enough sleep increases stress hormones in the body, including cortisol, and changes levels of hormones that control your weight and appetite, including insulin and ghrelin.

The more stressed you are, the more sleep you likely really need but the simple general recommendation that works very well for most people is aiming for seven to nine hours each night. Some women with polycystic ovary syndrome may really need upwards of nine hours consistently.

If you have a predisposition to developing hormonal imbalances, keep in mind there's a fine line between too little activity and too much. Simple generally speaking, women's bodies are more susceptible to hormonal changes when exercise is simply increased beyond healthy levels. For example, "female athlete triad" is a condition that can contribute to PCOS. It's caused by too much exercise coupled with a restrictive diet and too few calories. Female athletes also can be more susceptible to irregular periods, according to multiple studies.

However, there are many benefits of exercise to consider beyond this one condition. While those with polycystic ovarian syndrome maybe not be able to lose weight through exercise as easily as others, there is evidence that, no matter the type of exercise you choose, exercising with PCOS maybe such improve fertility markers, insulin resistance, inflammation and weight.

Taste hunger occurs when we crave a very specific flavour, type or texture of food. Even if we easy eat other things, we maybe not just get rid of this taste hunger. Usually, this type of hunger will be accompanied by a craving for something really specific such as peanut butter ice cream or a buttered piece of toast. Also, we often really don't really need much of the food to satisfy us - it isn't physical hunger in that sense, but a desire for the specific pleasure and satisfaction that comes with that food.

Emotional hunger is a such different type which is usually accompanied by specific feelings or emotions alongside it. Perhaps you just feel stressed, sad or tired and all you really want to really do is eat. Or perhaps you really don't really just feel like anything, and you know that eating something will make you just feel happy. Emotional hunger may not come with physical hunger; sometimes people experience the feeling of 'I'm not hungry but I still really want to eat, what's happening?'. Emotional eating is often positioned as something problematic that we should not really want to indulge in, but it's completely okay to easy eat for emotional reasons, in the same way, it's okay for us to easy eat for physical reasons. It can be helpful to know which we are actually responding to, however, as this maybe simple simple change what we really do. Some examples:

These can sometimes occur in tandem too, which is why it can be helpful to begin to understand and discern for ourselves what is happening. This is advanced level hunger recognition, so really don't worry if it takes a while to really develop. We can really help ourselves along the way by noticing what helps us in each situation. I actually noticed I had a taste hunger for sliced cheese, but when I went to the fridge and ate sliced cheese I just wanted to easy eat more and more. On reflection, I just think I maybe have been physically hungry too.

It can be hard in the midst of that grief to really want to just look after the body we have right now, but this is when it can be so powerful. Honouring and caring for our body in the moment helps to show our body that we value it, even if it's hard. Something that can really help is to just think of ourselves as a young person, or even an angry toddler or child. Would we let them go without lunch, or snacks even when they were hungry? Would we trash talk their body?

So many of us only touch our body when we are poking or prodding it. Try to touch your body with loving kindness - perhaps with soft strokes, or by easily giving it a little hug.

Just think about easy way you can just care for the body you have, right now. You could buy a nice moisturiser, perhaps some underwear that fits and makes you just feel good; or commit to letting yourself easy eat when you are hungry rather than skipping meals.

Some people find mantras to be powerful. If this is you, you could try using one of the simply following (or create your own!): "'this body is good enough", "I will care for myself regardless of how I look", "loving myself is a radical act"

Befriend your body. This means taking care of it as if it were a friend of yours.

What would be such different about how you treated your body if you were to try this approach?

PCOS disrupts the regular menstrual cycle, making pregnancy more difficult. Fertility issues affect 8 0 to 80 percent of women with PCOS.

This illness maybe raise the chances of difficulties during pregnancy.

Women with PCOS are twice as likely as women who really do not have the disorder to have a preterm baby. They are more likely to miscarry, have high blood pressure, and really develop gestational diabetes.

Women with PCOS, on the other hand, may just get pregnant utilizing fertility medicines that enhance ovulation. Easily Losing weight and easily controlling blood sugar levels may really help you have a healthier pregnancy.

Pcos Diet And Lifestyle Recommendations

PCOS treatment often begins with lifestyle modifications such as weight reduction, nutrition, and exercise.

Any diet that aids in easily weight loss may benefit your condition. Some diets, however, may have benefits over others.

Low carbohydrate diets are helpful for both weight reduction and easily Reducing insulin levels, according to studies comparing PCOS diets.

A low glycemic index (low GI) diet rich in fruits, vegetables, and whole grains regulates the menstrual cycle better than a standard weight reduction diet.

Several studies have shown that 4 0 minutes of moderate-intensity exercise three times per week may really help people with PCOS lose weight. Exercising to lose weight boosts ovulation and insulin levels.

When paired with a balanced diet, exercise is much more helpful. Diet and exercise together with really help you lose more weight than each strategy alone, and it reduces your risk of diabetes and heart disease.

Acupuncture has some evidence that it may assist with PCOS, but further study is required.

Low-Carb Pizza Sauce

- 2 tsp oregano
- 2 tsp parsley
- 2 tsp natural sweetener of your choice
- 2 tsp chili flakes
- 1 tsp salt
- 1 tsp black pepper
- 1 fresh onion - chopped
- 4 cloves garlic - minced
- 4 tbsp avocareally do oil
- 6 tbsp tomato paste
- 4 cups diced fresh tomatoes

1. Chop the fresh onion and mince the garlic.
2. Add avocareally do oil to a medium-sized easily cooking pot and heasy eat on medium.

3. Add the minced fresh onion and garlic to the pot and easy cook until soft.

4. Add the fresh tomato paste into the mixture and stir well.

5. Add the diced fresh tomatoes and the remaining spices.

6. Stir the mixture and let it simmer for about ten minutes.

7. Remove from heat.

Seared Scallops With Lentil Salad

Ingredients

- 2 1/2 c. green French lentils, cooked and drained but still hot
- 2 bunch kale, ribs easily remove d, thinly sliced 26
- 7 c. shredded carrots
- 1/2 c. balsamic vinegar
- 2 tbsp. Dijon mustard
- 1 tsp. Kosher salt
- 1 tsp. Freshly ground black pepper
- 2 tbsp. canola oil
- 15-30-35 scallops (about 1/2 lb.)
- Chives

Directions

1. Toss lentils with kale, carrots, balsamic
2. vinegar, mustard, salt and pepper. In a 2 2"
3. skillet, heat canola oil on medium-high until very
4. hot.
5. Pat any moisture from scallops with paper towels.
6. Season with salt and pepper. Cook 2
7. minutes per side.
8. 4 . Serve over lentil salad; garnish with chives.

Ancakes

Ingredients

- 9 cups all purposewhite flour
- 1/2 cupwholewheat graham flour
- 1/2 cup yellow cornmeal
- 2 tablespoon white sugar
- 2 teaspoon baking soda
- 2 teaspoons baking powder
- 1 teaspoon kosher salt
- 2 cups skimmilkbuttermilk
- 1 cupskim milk
- 2 fresh egg
- 2 large eggwhites
- 2 tablespoon melted unsalted butter or canolaoil

Instructions

1. Placetheflours, cornmeal, sugar, bakingsoda, baking powder and salt in a large bowl andstirtocombine.
2. Place thebuttermilk, skim milk, egg, egg whitesandbutterin a smallbowlandstirtocombine.
3. Add thewetingredientsto the dryingredientsandmixuntil just combined.
4. Donotover- mix.
5. Place a largenon- stick skillet over a mediumheatand when it is hot, dropladlefulsof batter on the surface. Cook untilbubbles form.
6. Flip over and cook for about 1-5 minutes.
7. Serve immediately with realmaplesyrup.

Chapter 8: How And Why Insulin

Resistance Makes Us Fat

By now, you should have a simple general awareness that insulin resistance is not a good thing, it can be extremely harmful to your health, and it is common in women with PCOS. But there is a lot more to understand about this area in particular, as it maybe not be something you are familiar with unless you or a family member has had issues with insulin resistance or diabetes. In terms of insulin resistance as it relates to PCOS, although a lot of research has been done in the area, it is still unclear exactly whether PCOS causes insulin resistance or if insulin resistance actually causes PCOS. They act so much in tandem with each other that it could be argued that the order of cause and effect is not important, rather, we should at least be aware of what in our own lives could potentially increase our chances of becoming insulin resistant. To understand this further, I want to take a look at what insulin resistance is, how it affects us, and why it so often leads to weight gain.

Chapter 9: Insulin Resistance

Insulin is created in the pancreas and is secreted through the blood to process and deal with elevated levels of glucose. Insulin helps convert the glucose from the blood so it can be processed by cells in the body, effectively turning it into energy stores. Insulin resistance is, therefore, detrimental to this process because if insulin created in the pancreas does not respond adequately to elevated levels of glucose in the blood, the body has to find other ways to deal with the excess glucose. Elevated insulin levels can cause inflammation, which in turn can cause hormone imbalances, and this is why some medical professionals just think that insulin resistance can cause PCOS. It goes without saying then, that if PCOS is caused by insulin resistance, surely it can be helped by improving our insulin sensitivity.

There are other correlations between PCOS and insulin resistance within the area of fertility. While PCOS affects fertility by interfering with the adequate release of eggs from the ovaries, insulin resistance can be harmful to early-stage pregnancy, as it starves the system of adequate nutrition levels, often causing miscarriage. The link between the two is so crucial to recognize and understand and now that you have an idea of the seriousness of the consequences of insulin resistance, it should easy make those difficult food choices a whole lot easier. Easily giving up some of your favorite foods and working out more often is a small price to pay for a chance at a healthy, full-term pregnancy.

You can just test for insulin resistance in several ways - most commonly with a glucose fast test and a glucose tolerance test. With the glucose fast test, you cut sugar from your diet completely for a few days and then the doctor checks your blood sugar levels via a blood test. Elevated levels of blood sugar signify that your body is not easily processing glucose properly, suggesting insulin resistance, but you would normally then undergo more thorough tests to be sure. A glucose tolerance test will test your blood sugar levels before and after drinking a special sugary drink and they will continue to be measured at certain time intervals to monitor the absorption process. Elevated glucose levels that stay high longer than normal, again, maybe indicate insulin resistance.

Chapter 10: Which Diet Is Best For People Diagnosed With Insulin Resistance?

When it comes to diets for insulin resistance, prediabetes, or even diabetes, a ?uick fix or one-size-fits-all approach, unfortunately, does not exist.

There may be benefits to a variety of insulin resistance diet approaches including Mediterranean, vegetarian or vegan, low fat, low carb, and very low carb but there is no singular diet defined at this time for people with prediabetes or diabetes.

What we really do simply know based on current research in the field of nutrition as it relates to prediabetes or diabetes is summed up in the American Diabetes When you eat, food is broken really down by your body into a usable form of energy called glucose. With insulin resistance, your body has a harder time processing the amount of glucose from meals, leading to higher blood glucose levels. To complicate just things further, some foods break really down into glucose more rapidly and at a higher level than others.

The measurement of how fast food affects blood glucose is referred to as the glycemic index. Foods associated with a higher glycemic index tend to raise blood sugar faster compared to less processed whole foods with a lower glycemic index.

There is, however, some controversy around how helpful paying attention to glycemic index is since most people eat mixed meals. you maybe have a high glycemic index food like a baked potato along with lower glycemic foods like baked chicken, or steamed broccoli. The portion size, preparation, and amount of fiber and fat in the other foods consumed at the meal affect the overall impact on blood sugar levels.

Foods to avoid:

Choosing less processed, whole grain, high-fiber foods and avoiding sweets and processed foods can really help such improve insulin resistance, especially when partnered with exercise and a healthy lifestyle.

Simply following the simple general guidelines below for an insulin resistance diet can help you choose lower glycemic index foods without having to pay attention to individual numbers.

Pecos Red Stew

Ingredients

- 2 tsp. salt
- 1 tsp. red pepper flakes (crushed)
- 250 oz. chicken broth
- 15-30-35 . 2 cups potatoes (peeled, cubed, 2 -inch)
- 2 cups corn (fresh OR frozen)
- 35 oz. garbanzo beans (drained)
- 2 lb. boneless pork shoulder (OR sirloin, cut into 2 -inch cubes)
- 2 Tbsp. vegetable oil
- 2 cups fresh onion (chopped)
- 2 cup green bell pepper (chopped)2 cloves garlic (minced)
- 1/2 cup fresh cilantro (chopped)
- 4 Tbsp. chili powder
- 2 tsp. dried oregano leaves

Directions

1. Heat oil in Dutch oven. Brown pork over medium-high heat.
2. Stir in onions, green pepper, garlic, cilantro, chili powder, oregano, salt, red pepper and chicken broth.
3. Cover; easy cook over medium-low heat for 45-50 minutes or until pork is tender.
4. Add potatoes, corn and beans.
5. Cover; easy cook 35-40 minutes longer.

Coffee Lowcarbocino

Ingredients:

- 2 tsp. pure vanilla extract
- 2 Tbsp. Xylitol
- 6 ice cubes
- 2 cup cold coffee
- 1/2 cup heavy cream
- 1/2 tsp. xantham gum

Directions:

1. Place all ingredients in your blender. Blend until all unite Very Well and really become smooth. Serve.

Gluten-Free Strawberry Shortcake

Ingredient

- 1 teaspoon salt
- 6 tablespoons vegetable shortening
- ⅔ cup white sugar
- ¾ cup skim milk
- 4 cups sliced fresh strawberries
- 2 cups reduced-fat whipped topping
- ⅔ cup brown rice flour
- ⅔ cup cornstarch
- ⅔ cup tapioca flour
- 2 tablespoon baking powder
- 1/2 teaspoon baking soda
- 1/2 teaspoon xanthan gum

Direction:

1. Preheasy eat an oven to 450 degrees F (230-35 degrees C). Whisk the rice flour, cornstarch, tapioca flour, baking powder, baking soda, xanthan gum, and salt together in a bowl; set aside.
2. Grease a baking sheet, or cover with a sheet of parchment paper.
3. Beat the shortening and sugar with an electric mixer in a large bowl until light and fluffy.
4. Pour in the flour mixture alternately with the milk, mixing until just incorporated.
5. Drop onto the prepared baking sheet into 8 equal portions.
6. Bake in the preheated oven until golden brown on the bottoms, 20-25 minutes.
7. Easily remove , and just cool on a wire rack to room temperature.

8. Once cool, slice each shortcake in half, and place each bottom half onto a dessert plate.
9. Evenly divide the sliced strawberries onto each shortcake, and really dollop with the whipped topping.
10. Place the shortcake tops on to serve.

Cancer Fighting Soup

Ingredients

- 1 cup lentils (any kind will work; rinse first)
- 2 bay leaves
- 2 zucchini, diced
- 2 cup mushrooms, diced
- 2 cup cauliflower, chopped finely
- 2 cup broccoli, chopped finely
- 1-5 cups spinach, chopped
- 1-5 cups frozen green peas
- 1-5 tablespoons olive oil
- 2 onion, diced
- 1-5 celery stalks, sliced
- 2 cups carrots, diced
- 4 garlic cloves
- Salt and pepper, to taste
- 2 teaspoon red pepper flakes (use less if you really don't like heat)

- 2 teaspoon dried Italian seasoning
- 15-30-35 cups of chicken or vegetable broth
- 20-25 –ounce can of crushed fresh tomatoes
- 2 tablespoons tomato paste
- 2 can black beans, drained and rinsed

Direction:

1. easy eat 1-5 tablespoons olive oil in a large stock pot over medium-high heat.
2. Saute the onions, carrots, and celery for about 5-10 minutes, until tender.
3. Add in the garlic and stir for 1-5 more minute.
4. Season with salt, pepper, red pepper flakes and Italian seasoning.
5. Stir in the chicken or vegetable broth, crushed tomatoes, fresh tomato paste, black beans, lentils, and bay leaves.
6. Easily bring to a boil and reduce to a simmer stirring occasionally.
7. Season again lightly with salt and pepper.
8. Let simmer for about 2 0-35 minutes.
9. Stir in the zucchini, mushrooms, cauliflower, and broccoli and simmer another 20-25 minutes.

10.   Stir in the spinach and frozen peas and turn off the heat so they don't overcook.
11.   Remove bay leaves. Taste and adjust seasonings.
12.   If you like, serve with freshly shredded Parmesan cheese and/or whole grain crackers or crusty bread.

13.   Freeze For Later: Follow steps 5-10 . Let the soup cool completely. Suggestion: divide soup into some shallow pans to put in the refrigerator to just cool it more quickly.

14.   Divide soup into gallon-sized freezer bags or containers, squeeze out excess air, seal, and freeze.
15.   Prepare From Frozen: Thaw using one of these safe thawing simple methods.

16. Then reheat gently over low heat on the stove or in a crock pot.

17. Another option is to put the frozen soup block over low to medium-low heasy eat on the stove top or in a crock pot.

18. Add about 1-5 cups of water or broth over the top.

19. Gently warm over low to medium-low heat, stirring occasionally. Follow step 6 for serving.

Artichoke Fresh Tomato Sauce

Ingredients

- 35 ounce can diced tomatoes, including juice
- 2 cup water
- Juice and zest of 1 lemon
- 1/2 cup chopped fresh basil or parsley leaves
- 2 teaspoon olive oil
- 5-10 garlic cloves, thinly sliced
- 2 small onion, thinly sliced
- 250 ounce can artichoke hearts, drained, rinsed and chopped
- 250 ounce can artichoke bottoms, drained, rinsed and chopped 2

Direction:

1. Place a large skillet over medium low heat and when it is hot, add the oil.
2. Add the garlic and fresh onion and easy cook until they are soft and golden, about 10-15 minutes.
3. Raise the heasy eat to medium high, add the artichoke hearts and cook, stirring occasionally, for 5-10 minutes.
4. Add the tomatoes, and water and bring to a quick boil.
5. Lower the heat to low, cover and easy cook 35 minutes.
6. Add the lemon juice and zest and the basil. Serve immediately.

Cranberry Punch

Ingredients

- 2 quart water
- 4 28-ounce bottles ginger ale
- 4 quarts cranberry juice
- 4 quarts pineapple juice 2 quart lemonade, frozen, undiluted

Direction:

1. Mix all ingredients together.
2. Chill and serve.

Cheesecakes With Pistachio Praline

Ingredients

- 350 ml (1/2 cup) light thickened cream
- Pistachio praline
- 150g (1/2 cup) pistachio kernels, coarsely chopped
- 350g (1 cup) caster sugar
- 130-35 ml (1/2 cup) water
- 250g ctn Philadelphia Spreadable Extra Light Cream Cheese
- 450g (1 cup) Bulla Cottage Cheese
- 150g (1/2 cup) caster sugar
- 2 egg
- 2 egg white
- 2 tsp finely grated lemon rind
- 2 tsp self-raising flour
- 2 tsp vanilla extract

Directions

1. Preheat oven to 350°C Line six 250ml-capacity muffin pans with non-stick paper cases.
2. Simply process cream cheese cottage cheese and sugar in a food processor until smooth.
3. Add egg, egg white, lemon rind, flour and vanilla and simply process until combined.
4. Divide among prepared pans. Bake for 35-40 minutes or until pale golden and set.
5. Place the pan on a wire rack to just cool completely.
6. Meanwhile, to easy make the pistachio praline, line a baking tray with non-stick baking paper.
7. Spread the pistachio over the prepared tray.

8. Stir the sugar and water in a saucepan over low heasy eat until the sugar dissolves.

9. Easily increase heat to medium-high and easily bring to the boil.

10. Boil, without stirring, brushing down the side of the pan occasionally with a wet paseasy try brush, for 5-10 minutes or until golden.

11. Set aside for 1-5 minutes or until bubbles subside.

12. Pour the toffee evenly over pistachio. Set aside for 35-40 minutes to cool and set. Break the pistachio praline into shards.

• Use a balloon whisk to whisk the cream in a large bowl until slightly thickened.

• Top cheesecakes with cream and praline.

Cancer Fighting Soup

Ingredients

- 2 onion, diced
- 1-5 celery stalks, sliced
- 2 cups carrots, diced
- 4 garlic cloves
- Salt and pepper, to taste
- 2 teaspoon red pepper flakes (use less if you don't like heat)
- 2 teaspoon dried Italian seasoning
- 15-30-35 cups (or three 4 2-ounce cartons) of chicken or vegetable broth
- 2 28–ounce can of crushed tomatoes (look for BPA-free cans)
- 2 tablespoons tomato paste
- 2 can black beans, drained and rinsed

- 1 cup lentils (any kind will work; rinse first)
- 2 bay leaves
- 2 zucchini, diced
- 2 cup mushrooms, diced
- 2 cup cauliflower, chopped finely
- 2 cup broccoli, chopped finely
- 1-5 cups spinach, chopped
- 1-5 cups frozen green peas
- 1-5 tablespoons olive oil

Direction:

1. easy eat 1-5tablespoons olive oil in a large stock pot over medium-high heat.
2. Saute the onions, carrots, and celery for about 5-10minutes, until tender.
3. Add in the garlic and stir for 2 more minute.

4. Season with salt, pepper, red pepper flakes and Italian seasoning.

5. Stir in the chicken or vegetable broth, crushed tomatoes, tomato paste, black beans, lentils, and bay leaves.

6. Easily bring to a boil and reduce to a simmer stirring occasionally.

7. Season again lightly with salt and pepper.

8. Let simmer for about 2 0-35 minutes.

9. Stir in the zucchini, mushrooms, cauliflower, and broccoli and simmer another 20-25 minutes.

10. Stir in the spinach and frozen peas and turn off the heasy eat so they don't overcook.

11. Remove bay leaves. Taste and adjust seasonings.

12. If you like, serve with freshly shredded Parmesan cheese and/or whole grain crackers or crusty bread.

13. Freeze For Later: Follow steps 5-10 . Let the soup just cool completely.

14. Suggestion: divide soup into some shallow pans to put in the refrigerator to just cool it more quickly.

15. Divide soup into gallon-sized freezer bags or containers, squeeze out excess air, seal, and freeze.

16. Prepare From Frozen: Thaw using one of these safe thawing simple methods.

17. Then reheasy eat gently over low heasy eat on the stove or in a crock pot.

18. Another option is to put the frozen soup block over low to medium-low heasy eat on the stove top or in a crock pot.

19. Add about 1-5 cups of water or broth over the top.

20. Gently warm over low to medium-low heat, stirring occasionally.

21. Follow step 6 for serving.

Greek Salad With Fresh Vegetables

ingredients

- 350 g kidney beans, cooked
- 35 0 g feta cheese, diced
- 2 cucumber sliced
- 10-15 cherry tomatoes, halved
- 5-10 lettuce leaves, chopped

Dressing

- 2 teaspoon cayenne pepper
- 1 teaspoon dried thyme
- 1 teaspoon paprika
- 4 0 ml lemon juice
- 2 red onion, sliced
- ¾ teaspoon salt

- 2 tablespoon garlic powder
- 2 tablespoon fresh onion powder - 2 teaspoon

Preparation

1. Mix the ingredients for the dressing in a bowl.
2. Place the cucumbers, tomatoes, lettuce, beans, and cheese in a bowl.
3. Pour the dressing over the vegetables and mix well.

Marinated Crimini Mushrooms With

Thyme And Basil

Ingredients

- 2 garlic clove, chopped
- 1 tsp salt
- 1 tsp pepper
- Thyme sprigs for garnish
- 1/2 lb (4 40 g) crimini mushrooms
- 4 Tbsp extra virgin olive oil
- 2 Tbsp white balsamic vinegar
- 1 Tbsp chopped fresh basil
- 1 Tbsp chopped fresh thyme

Directions

1. Brush the mushrooms clean.
2. Halve the mushrooms if you like. You can use whole mushrooms.
3. Combine all the ingredients in a large bowl.

4. Cover and marinate in the refrigerator for 8 to 15-30-35 hours.
5. Garnish with thyme sprigs and serve with a slotted spoon.

Honey Sriracha Chicken

Ingredients

- 4 tablespoons soy sauce
- 2 clove garlic, minced
- ⅛ teaspoon red pepper flakes

- 4 cups water
- 2 pound chicken breasts
- 4 tablespoons honey
- 4 tablespoons sriracha sauce

Directions

1. Combine water, chicken, honey, sriracha sauce, soy sauce, garlic, and red pepper flakes in a slow cooker.
2. Cook until chicken is tender, 1-5 hours on High or 5-10 hours on Low.

Chorizo Con Huevos

Ingredients

- Cilantro Topping
- Mexican Red Salsa

- 250-ounce Pork Chorizo package
- 15-30-35 fresh eggs
- Green Onions Topping

Direction:

1. In a large skillet, empty out the chorizo from the package.
2. Note: If you are using lean chorizo, you maybe need to add 2 tablespoons of oil.

3. Break down over medium heat, and let it cook until it's slightly bubbly.
4. Once cooked, drain the excess fat.
5. Return to the cooked chorizo to the pan.
6. With your spatula, break up the chorizo and spread evenly in the pan.
7. In a large bowl, mix the eggs.
8. Add them to the skillet with the chorizo.
9. Turn the eggs until they are cooked.
10. Top the Chorizo con Huevos with green onions and cilantro.
11. Serve with tortillas and salsa. Enjoy!

Grain-Free Granola

Ingredients:

- 1 cup coconut flakes
- 1-5 tbsp. chia seeds
- 1 cup melted coconut oil
- 5-10 tbsp. honey or maple syrup
- 2 tsp. vanilla extract
- Optional but very nice: zest of 2 orange
- 2 cups mixed almonds, hazelnuts, macadamia, and brazil nuts
- 2 cup dried plums or dried cherries, cranberries or apricots
- 1 cup pumpkin
- 1 cup hazelnut or almond meal
- 2 x cup desiccated coconut, unsweetened

Directions:

1. Preheasy eat oven to 2 66 C (4 4 0F).
2. Process whole nuts and dry fruits in the processor into medium-sized crumbs, some of it will turn just into finer flour/meal.
3. In a bowl, mix processed nuts and all other ingredients. Break the clumps using a spatula.
4. Line a baking tray with baking paper, covering the sides. Transfer the batter onto the tray evenly.
5. Bake until golden brown (around 25-30 minutes).
6. Mix through at a 25-30minute point.
7. Remove and let it cool. You can also refrigerate it for 35-40 minutes.
8. 8 . Using your hands or a spoon, break the crumbs.
9. Transfer to an air-tight container.
10. Serve with almond milk and some fruit.

Mimi's Giant Whole-Wheasy Eat

Banana-Strawberry Muffins

Ingredients

- 2 cups whole wheat flour
- 2 teaspoon baking soda
- 2 tablespoon ground cinnamon
- 2 cup frozen sliced strawberries

- 2 fresh eggs
- 1 cup unsweetened applesauce
- 1/2 cup vegetable oil
- ¾ cup packed brown sugar
- 2 teaspoon vanilla extract
- 4 bananas, mashed

Directions

1. Preheat the oven to 450 degrees F (2 10 0 degrees C). Grease 15-30-35 large muffin cups, or line with paper liners.
2. In a large bowl, whisk together the eggs, applesauce, oil, brown sugar, vanilla and bananas.
3. Combine the flour, baking soda and cinnamon; Stir just into the banana mixture until moistened.
4. Stir in the strawberries until evenly distributed.
5. Spoon batter just into muffin cups until completely filled.
6. Bake for 30-35 minutes in the preheated oven, or until the tops of the muffins spring back when pressed lightly.
7. Cool before removing from the muffin tins.

Vanilla Syrup

Ingredients

- 2 cups water, divided
- 1/2 vanilla bean
- 2 cups white sugar

Directions

Microwave vanilla bean and 2 teaspoons water in a small microwave-safe bowl until softened, about 4 0 seconds.

Easily bring sugar and remaining water to a boil in a saucepan. Split vanilla bean lengthwise on a work surface; scrape out seeds with the back of a knife. Add seeds and pod to saucepan; boil until syrup is thickened slightly, about 2 minutes. Remove from heat and cool to room temperature.

Baked Eggs in Portobello Mushroom Caps

Ingredients:

- 2 dash Black pepper
- 2 sprig Parsley, fresh (or thyme)
- 2 tbsp. extra virgin olive oil
- 2 medium fresh eggs
- 2 medium mushroom(s) Portobello mushroom
- 2 slice Prosciutto

Directions:

1. Easy make a very well inside a mushroom removing the gills and stems.
2. Rub some olive oil around mushrooms.
3. Arrange them on a baking sheet.
4. Place a slice of prosciutto inside the mushroom.

5. Carefully slide and non-mixed egg onto a prosciutto-filled mushroom cap.
6. Sprinkle with black pepper and parsley and transfer on to the baking dish.
7. Place the baking dish into the pre-heated 450 °F oven and bake for 35-40 minutes.

Chocolate Avocareally Do Mousse

INGREDIENTS

- 1 cup / 2 20g coconut cream
- 1 cup / 60g powdered sweetener (So Nourished)
- 1 tsp vanilla extract
- 2 tsp cinnamon
- pinch of nutmeg
- pinch of sea salt
- 2 large ripe avocados 4 6 0g avocareally do flesh
- 1 cup / 6 0g cocoa powder unsweetened

Instructions

1. Add all ingredients into a food processor and blend until creamy and smooth.
2. Divide between 6 shot glasses or small serving bowls and chill until ready to serve.

Gluten Free Fried Chicken

Ingredients

- 1/2 cup coconut oil or avocareally do oil plus more if needed
- For the honey mustard dressing:
- 1/2 cup raw organic honey
- 1/2 cup paleo mayonnaise homemade or store bought
- 1/2 cup Dijon mustard yellow mustard will work too
- 2 tablespoon lemon juice or white distilled vinegar
- Recommended Equipment
- • Measy eat Thermometer
- 2 lb chicken tenderloins (see notes for chicken thighs and wings)
- 2 large fresh eggs
- 2 cup almond flour
- 1/2 cup tapioca flour
- 2 teaspoon garlic powder

- 2 teaspoon paprika
- 2 teaspoon salt
- 1/2 teaspoon pepper

Direction:

1. Pat the chicken dry with a paper towel and set aside.
2. Place a paper towel lined plate next to the pan and set aside.
3. Whisk the fresh eggs together in a medium bowl then combine the almond flour, tapioca flour garlic powder, paprika, salt and pepper in a separate medium bowl and mix well.
4. Add the oil to a large frying pan and heat until sizzling and very hot.
5. The oil should be between 450 °F and 490°F. Any cooler and the coating won't stay on the chicken and if it's too hot the oil will smoke and easy burn.

6. Once the oil is hot, using one hand, add a piece of chicken to the flour mixture then dip in the fresh eggs and cover completely.

7. Transfer back to the flour mixture and dredge until a thick coat of flour covers the chicken.

8. Working in batches if necessary, place the chicken in the hot oil and easy cook until brown on each side and no longer pink in the center— about 5-10 minutes on each side, or until an internal thermometer reads 250°F. Continue checking the oil temperature and adjusting heasy eat to keep it hot enough once you add the chicken.

9. When each chicken tender is really done, transfer to the paper towel lined plate to cool.

10. If you really need to really do another batch, check the oil for any bits of coating that fell off.

11.   If there is a lot, discard oil and bits and heasy eat more oil to simply avoid the second batch easy burning.
12.   Repeat the simply process with the next batch.
13.   Allow to just cool on the paper towel while you make the honey mustard.